12 Week Exercise Program:

Full Body Weight & Free Weights Workout

Designed by: Elaine G Workouts SA

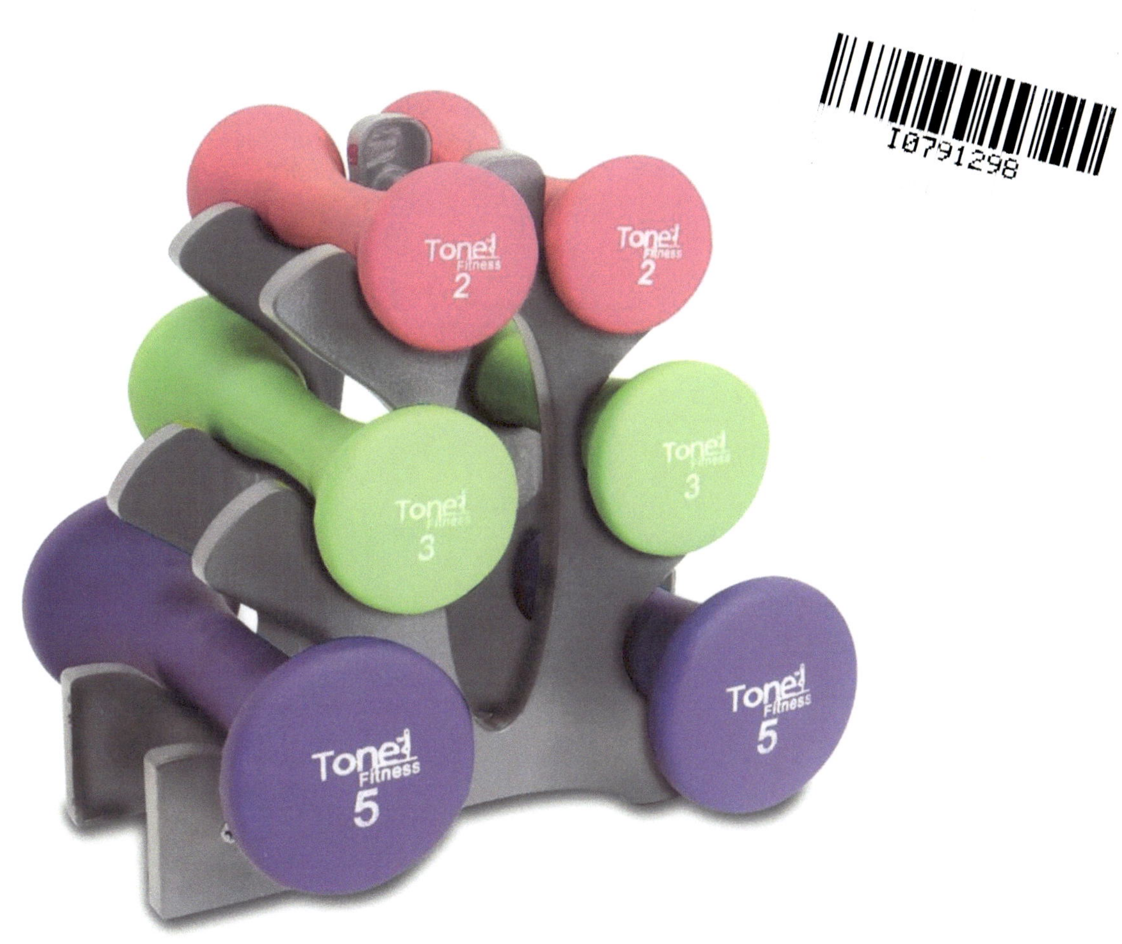

Disclaimer

The information contained in this book is made available to you as a self-help tool
for your own use. The use of this information should be based on your own due
diligence and you agree that this program is not liable for any success or failure of your
physique that is directly or indirectly related to the purchase and use of this information.
It is strongly recommended that you consult with your Doctor before beginning any
exercise program. You should be in good physical condition and be able to participate
in the exercise. You should understand that when participating in any exercise or
exercise program, there is the possibility of physical injury. If you engage in this
exercise program, you agree that you do so at your own risk, are voluntarily
participating in these activities, and assuming all risk of injury to yourself.
The information provided is based on personal and professional experience
designed by a qualified fitness trainer who has a Diploma in Personal Training
obtained through TriFocus Fitness Academy in South Africa.

Contents

Introduction

Hello there,

Thank you for purchasing my workouts. My name is El, I am a qualified Personal Fitness Trainer and I am here to bring to you, personally, workouts that you can do in the privacy of your home or in the gym, whichever you feel best that works for you. This training manual does not have lots of pages that are filled with diet, nutrition and other scientific jargon is written in most workout books, which means I am going to be getting to the complete workouts in a very few short pages.

With that being said and I would not be doing my job if I did not mention this… I am a certified nutritionist as well, however, I will not be telling you to follow any specific lifestyle program. The market is flooded with so much information on what to eat and what not to eat, that I will not add to it. What I will recommend is **MINDFUL EATING.** Think before you put that chocolate, cake or bread in your mouth, sure go ahead and eat it, it's just going to take you longer to get fit and become healthy, lose fat or whatever your goal is here. You will be letting yourself down. Remember, you purchased this workout for a reason!

Please bear in mind though, if you want to improve your performance, change your body shape, lose fat or want to accelerate and optimize your physical activity, please do follow a healthy lifestyle. Yes, you can lose weight with diet alone, but exercise is an important component, that is why you bought my book is it not? Thank you! Without it, only a portion of your weight loss is from fat — you're also stripping away muscle and bone density. As a rule of thumb, weight loss is generally 75 percent diet and 25 percent exercise.
I do firmly believe in calories in, calories out and there are a lot of diet apps for you to choose from that will calculate your daily calorie intake for fat loss. Examples are Fat Secret, MyFitnessPal and Yazio.

Dieting and exercising should not be hard and complicated as life in general is complicated enough as it is.

DISCIPLINE AND DEDICATION – IT WILL BECOME A PART OF YOU IF YOU WANT IT BAD ENOUGH!

About these workouts

These 36 complete workouts consist of full body weight and free weights, done 3 days per week, and should not take you more than 1 hour per day. If you do not have any specific equipment at home to do these workout, and are a beginner, you can make use of 500ml water bottles or canned foods for arm exercises, your stairs at home for step ups, and even you chairs for one leg get ups and Bulgarian squats and your couch for V-ups if you need something to sit on. If you are a gym goer, and want to take this program along with, you can modify the equipment you use and go for the machines for some of the exercises or just stay in the functional fitness part of the gym.

If you would like to invest in some home equipment, I would highly recommend that the first thing you buy is a pair of 2kg wrist weights. These are magic weights to have as you can use them to increase your weights when you want to go up sizes in dumbbells. For instance, if you start off with 1kg dumbbells, and they feel too light for you, add the 2 kg wrist weights and you immediately have 3kg weights on each arm, and then the next set of dumbbells you can buy is the 3kg, add the 2 kg wrist weight and you have 5kg weights per side. If you start with the 2 kg wrist weights and want to increase your weights, you can buy 2 kg barbells and you immediately have 4kg weights to work with. You see where I am going with this here? Other equipment recommend would be dumbbells, an ab-wheel, a stepper (maybe an adjustable one, because as you get stronger you will be able to step higher) and a barbell with added weights. A bit later on in the weeks as you progress, you will need a bench but it's not necessary as some of the bench exercises can be done in standing position or lying on the floor if your budget is a bit tight.

If you are not sure of form when you do the exercises or not sure of the exercises themselves, please go ahead and YouTube the exercises as there are plenty of videos explaining form and movement.

Why these workouts?

WHY am I bringing these workouts to you? Not everyone can afford gym memberships and/or a personal trainer or you have a gym membership, but you have no idea what to do, so you head to the cardio section and stay there as long as possible before you get bored...I know, I have been there and done that...it's kind of sucks! Now I have a personal gym at home and I have people joining me for one on one sessions, who are using these exact same workouts.

These workouts are for losing fat, body and muscle shaping and toning but you are encouraged to do cardio on alternate days for 30 minutes, even if it's just walking. These are exercises that will help you with everyday movements, like getting up from a chair, bending to pick up our precious babies or the mess they make all over the house. These exercises can be done by male, female, seniors and youngsters who are healthy.

My goal with this program is to simplify the process rather than complicate it. This program will have some challenges for you, some exercises won't necessarily feel "easy" but they will be simple. This program is practical and it should fit easily into a busy modern day lifestyle. I fully believe that you can have the body you want without having to sacrifice your social life to get it.

About the exercises, reps and sets:

If this is the only workout program you purchase for yourself, then there are ways to progress and challenge yourself without changing the exercises. I would recommend that you finish the first 12 weeks in their order, with the reps and sets given, if you are a beginner. Thereafter, you can swop any week and day around, increase your reps to suit your new found strength, and even lessen the rest period and move through the exercises quicker for a bit more of a cardio/ HIIT session.

Lactic acid build-up and soreness after a workout:

The 2nd and 3rd day after your workout, you will most probably feel sore, this is quite normal. Lactic acid build up due to exercise is usually temporary and not cause for a lot of concern, it can affect your workouts by causing discomfort BUT you need to do that workout on the third day, no matter how sore you are, do not let that discomfort stop you! The best way to work that soreness away is YES! Doing a workout. I promise you, it works. This is how you know that you have actually worked your muscles. I can recommend that you drink a glass of alkaline powder in water after a workout, before you go to bed at night and a glass in the morning. Not only does it alleviate some of the lactic acid build up but it does have other benefits on the body as well.

PLEASE DITCH THE SCALE….if you don't want to, that's up to you but do take body measurements in conjunction with your scale reading as I can promise you one thing…your centimetre or inches lost is the best indication of these workouts doing what they should be doing, if you are consistent, putting in the work and following a mindful eating approach.
Muscle weighs more than fat so as you lose the fat, the more dense heavier muscle is forming. Rather go by how your clothes fit your body and you will possibly even go out and buy a new wardrobe.

Ok, can we get to the workouts already? I love this part!

- 12 weeks of full body workouts consisting of your own body weight and free weights.
- 36 workouts.
- 3 days per week, less than 1 hour each, for 3 months.
- Workouts progress during the following weeks.
- Choose a time that is best suited for you to exercise.
- Mark your workouts off on a calendar or get yourself a fitness journal and tracker.
- You should start to notice a difference in body composition from 6 weeks.
- Practice **MINDFUL EATING!** (calories in, calories out)
- **DISCIPLINE AND DEDICATION!**
- **Ways to progress:**
  Same weight **more reps**   Same weight **more sets**   Same reps **more weight**
- **Per side** means each leg or arm or side must do the same amount of reps as the other.
- **Take body measurements**

You've got this!

Get ready to transform your life mentally and physically!

NB: Please do take care and if you cannot finish all 3 sets, that's ok! As you get stronger you will be able to finish every workout. This is not a race to the finish line, this is a lifestyle, be consistent, be disciplined and you will be well on your way to a healthier and fitter life.

Body weight and strength training

Week 1 Day 1

Exercise	Reps	Sets	Rest
Goblet squats with dumbbells	10	3	1 min
Curtsy lunge (without dumbbells)	10 per side	3	1 min
Dumbbell Shoulder press	10	3	1 min
Rest 60 seconds then repeat above exercises for 3 rounds.			
Tri-cep dips or overhead tri-cep extensions with dumbbells	10	3	1 min
Push ups	10	3	1 min
Elbow or straight arm plank	60 seconds	3	1 min
Rest 60 seconds then repeat above exercises for 3 rounds.			
One arm dumbbell row	10	3	1 min
T-Bend	10 per side	3	1 min
Squat and lateral arm raise with dumbbells	10	3	1 min
Rest 60 seconds then repeat above exercises for 3 rounds.			

Body weight and strength training

Week 1 Day 2

Exercise	Reps	Sets	Rest
Curtsy lunge (without dumbbells)	10 per side	3	1 min
Dumbbell shoulder press	10	3	1 min
Front arm raises with dumbbells	10	3	1 min
Rest 60 seconds then repeat above exercises for 3 rounds.			
T-Bend	10 per side	3	1 min
Squat and lateral arm raise with dumbbells	10	3	1 min
One arm dumbbell row	10 per side	3	1 min
Rest 60 seconds then repeat above exercises for 3 rounds.			
Dumbbell squat	10	3	1 min
Russian Twist (with or without weights)	10 per side	3	1 min
Tri-cep dips or overhead tri-cep extensions with dumbbells	10	3	1 min
Rest 60 seconds then repeat above exercises for 3 rounds.			

Body weight and strength training

Week 1 Day 3

Exercise	Reps	Sets	Rest
T-Bend	10 per side	3	1 min
Tri-cep dips or overhead tri-cep extensions with dumbbells	10	3	1 min
Curtsy lunge (without dumbbells)	10 per side	3	1 min
Rest 60 seconds then repeat above exercises for 3 rounds.			
Step ups	10 per side	3	1 min
Alternate dumbbell front and lateral arm raises	10 each	3	1 min
Stiff leg deadlift (with barbell or dumbbells)	10	3	1 min
Rest 60 seconds then repeat above exercises for 3 rounds.			
Russian Twist (with or without weights)	10 per side	3	1 min
Dumbbell row and kickback	10	3	1 min
Dumbbell squat	10	3	1 min
Rest 60 seconds then repeat above exercises for 3 rounds.			

Body weight and strength training

Week 2 Day 1

Exercise	Reps	Sets	Rest
Push ups	10	3	1 min
Bent dumbbell row	10	3	1 min
Upright dumbbell row	10	3	1 min
Rest 60 seconds then repeat above exercises for 3 rounds.			
Reverse lunge	10 per side	3	1 min
Stiff leg deadlift (with barbell or dumbbells)	10	3	1 min
Bulgarian split squat (use a bench or chair seat)	10 per side	3	1 min
Rest 60 seconds then repeat above exercises for 3 rounds.			
Elbow or straight arm plank	60 seconds	3	1 min
Mountain climbers	10 per side	3	1 min
V-Ups	10	3	1 min
Rest 60 seconds then repeat above exercises for 3 rounds.			

Body weight and strength training

Week 2 Day 2

Exercise	Reps	Sets	Rest
Dumbbell squat	10	3	1 min
Reverse lunges	10 per side	3	1 min
Stiff leg deadlift (with barbell or dumbbells)	10	3	1 min
Rest 60 seconds then repeat above exercises for 3 rounds.			
Step ups	10 per side	3	1 min
Elbow or straight arm plank	60 seconds	3	1 min
Mountain climbers	10 per side	3	1 min
Rest 60 seconds then repeat above exercises for 3 rounds.			
Bicep curl and shoulder press	10	3	1 min
Push ups	10	3	1 min
Bent dumbbell row	10	3	1 min
Rest 60 seconds then repeat above exercises for 3 rounds.			

Body weight and strength training

Week 2 Day 3

Exercise	Reps	Sets	Rest
T-Bend	10 per side	3	1 min
Dumbbell Shoulder press	10	3	1 min
Side plank (on elbow or straight arm)	30 sec per side	3	1 min
Rest 60 seconds then repeat above exercises for 3 rounds.			
One arm dumbbell row	10 per side	3	1 min
Dumbbell Bicep curl and shoulder press	10	3	1 min
Push ups	10	3	1 min
Rest 60 seconds then repeat above exercises for 3 rounds.			
Curtsy lunge (with or without dumbbells)	10 per side	3	1 min
Goblet squat with dumbbell	10	3	1 min
Reverse lunge or walking lunges	10 per side	3	1 min
Rest 60 seconds then repeat above exercises for 3 rounds.			

Body weight and strength training

Week 3 Day 1

Exercise	Reps	Sets	Rest
Push ups	10	3	1 min
One leg get ups (use a bench or chair seat)	10 per side	3	1 min
Cross over abdominal crunch	10 per side	3	1 min
Rest 60 seconds then repeat above exercises for 3 rounds.			
Bent over Dumbbell row and kickback	10	3	1 min
Goblet squat with dumbbell	10	3	1 min
Dumbbell shoulder press	10	3	1 min
Rest 60 seconds then repeat above exercises for 3 rounds.			
Alternating dumbbell bicep curl and hammer curl	10 of each	3	1 min
T-Bend	10 per side	3	1 min
Mountain climbers	10 per side	3	1 min
Rest 60 seconds then repeat above exercises for 3 rounds.			

Body weight and strength training

Week 3 Day 2

Exercise	Reps	Sets	Rest
T-Bend	10	3	1 min
Dumbbell row and kickback	10	3	1 min
Bulgarian split squat (use a bench or chair seat)	10 per side	3	1 min
Rest 60 seconds then repeat above exercises for 3 rounds.			
Reverse lunge or walking lunges	10 per side	3	1 min
Tri-cep dips or overhead tri-cep extensions with dumbbells	10	3	`1 min
Stiff leg deadlift (with barbell or dumbbells)	10	3	1 min
Rest 60 seconds then repeat above exercises for 3 rounds.			
V-ups	10	3	1 min
Dumbbell bi-cep curl and shoulder press	10	3	1 min
Goblet squat with dumbbell	10	3	1 min
Rest 60 seconds then repeat above exercises for 3 rounds.			

Body weight and strength training

Week 3 Day 3

Exercise	Reps	Sets	Rest
Goblet squat	10	3	1 min
Mountain climbers	10 per side	3	1 min
Tri-cep dips or overhead tri-cep extensions with dumbbells	10	3	1 min
Rest 60 seconds then repeat above exercises for 3 rounds.			
Stiff leg deadlifts (with barbell or dumbbell)	10	3	1 min
Elbow or straight arm planks	60 seconds	3	1 min
Dumbbell hammer curl and bicep curl	10	3	1 min
Rest 60 seconds then repeat above exercises for 3 rounds.			
One leg get-ups	10 per side	3	1 min
T-bend	10	3	1 min
One arm dumbbell row	10 per side	3	1 min
Rest 60 seconds then repeat above exercises for 3 rounds.			

Body weight and strength training

Week 4 Day 1

Exercise	Reps	Sets	Rest
Push ups	10	3	1 min
Curtsy lunge (without dumbbells)	10 per side	3	1 min
Step ups	10 per side	3	1 min
Dumbbell shoulder press	10	3	1 min
Bent dumbbell row	10	3	1 min
Dumbbell squat	10	3	1 min
Abdominal side crunches	10 per side	3	1 min
Dumbbell front and lateral arm raises	10 of each	3	1 min
Bulgarian split squat (use a bench or chair seat)	10 per side	3	1 min
Elbow or straight arm Plank	60 seconds	3	1 min
Rest 60 seconds then repeat above exercises for 3 rounds.			

Body weight and strength training

Week 4 Day 2

Exercise	Reps	Sets	Rest
Curtsy lunge	10 per side	3	1 min
Abdominal crunches	10	3	1 min
Tri-cep dips or overhead tri-cep extensions with dumbbells	10	3	1 min
Stiff leg deadlift (with barbell or dumbbells)	10 per side	3	1 min
Russian twists (with or without weight)	10 per side	3	1 min
Dumbbell shoulder press	10	3	1 min
Bent dumbbell row	10	3	1 min
Goblet squat with dumbbell	10	3	1 min
Step ups	10 per side	3	1 min
Dumbbell front and lateral arm raises	10 each	3	1 min
Rest 60 seconds then repeat above exercises for 3 rounds.			

Body weight and strength training

Week 4 Day 3

Exercise	Reps	Sets	Rest
Goblet squat with dumbbell	10	3	1 min
Tri-cep dips or overhead tri-cep extensions with dumbbells	10	3	1 min
Walking lunges	10 per side	3	1 min
Abdominal side crunches	10 per side	3	1 min
Dumbbell lateral arm raises	10	3	1 min
Stiff leg deadlift (with barbell or dumbbells)	10	3	1 min
Mountain climbers	10 per side	3	1 min
One arm dumbbell press	10 per side	3	1 min
V-ups	10	3	1 min
Up Right dumbbell row	10	3	1 min
Rest 60 seconds then repeat above exercises for 3 rounds.			

Body weight and strength training

Week 5 Day 1   (Exercises progress)

Exercise	Reps	Sets	Rest
Push ups	12	3	1 min
Curtsy lunge (with dumbbells)	10 per side	3	1 min
Step ups	10	3	1 min
Dumbbell shoulder press	10	3	1 min
Tri-cep dips or overhead tri-cep extensions with dumbbells	12	3	1 min
Goblet squat with dumbbell	10	3	1 min
Elbow or straight arm plank	70 seconds	3	1 min
One arm dumbbell row	10 per side	3	1 min
T-Bend	10 per side	3	1 min
Squat and lateral arm raise with dumbbells	10	3	1 min
Rest 60 seconds then repeat above exercises for 3 rounds.			

Body weight and strength training

Week 5 Day 2

Exercise	Reps	Sets	Rest
Curtsy lunge (with dumbbells)	10 per side	3	1 min
Step ups	10	3	1 min
Dumbbell front arm raises	10	3	1 min
T-Bend	10	3	1 min
Squat and lateral arm raise with dumbbells	10	3	1 min
Bent over dumbbell row	10	3	1 min
Dumbbell squat	10	3	1 min
Dumbbell Shoulder press	10	3	1 min
Elbow or straight arm side plank	30 secs per side	3	1 min
Tri-cep dips or overhead tri-cep extensions with dumbbells	12	3	1 min
Rest 60 seconds then repeat above exercises for 3 rounds.			

Body weight and strength training

Week 5 Day 3

Exercise	Reps	Sets	Rest
T-Bend	10	3	1 min
Tri-cep dips or overhead tri-cep extensions with dumbbells	12	3	1 min
Curtsy lunge (with dumbbells)	10	3	1 min
Stiff leg deadlift (with barbell or dumbbells)	10	3	1 min
Dumbbell Front and lateral arm raises	10 each	3	1 min
Upright Row with (barbell or dumbbells)	10	3	1 min
Elbow or straight arm plank	70 seconds	3	1 min
Bent over dumbbell arm rows and kickbacks	10	3	1 min
Dumbbell squat	10	3	1 min
One leg get ups (use bench or chair seat)	10 per side	3	1 min
Rest 60 seconds then repeat above exercises for 3 rounds.			

Body weight and strength training

Week 6 Day 1

Exercise	Reps	Sets	Rest
Push ups	12	3	1 min
Bent dumbbell row	12	3	1 min
Flat bench press with dumbbell	10	3	1 min
Rest 60 seconds then repeat above exercises for 3 rounds.			
Walking lunges with dumbbells	12 per side	3	1 min
Stiff leg deadlift	10	3	1 min
Bulgarian split squat (use a bench or chair)	10 per side	3	1 min
Rest 60 seconds then repeat above exercises for 3 rounds.			
Elbow or straight arm plank	75 seconds	3	1 min
Standing dumbbell oblique side crunches	12 per side	3	1 min
Squat and dumbbell shoulder press	10	3	1 min
Rest 60 seconds then repeat above exercises for 3 rounds.			

Body weight and strength training

Week 6 Day 2

Exercise	Reps	Sets	Rest
Goblet squat	10	3	1 min
One leg get ups (use a bench or chair)	10 per side	3	1 min
Stiff leg deadlift with barbell or dumbbells	10	3	1 min
Rest 60 seconds then repeat above exercises for 3 rounds.			
Step ups with dumbbells	12 per side	3	1 min
Elbow or straight arm plank	75 seconds	3	1 min
Lying cross over abdominal crunch	12 per side	3	1 min
Rest 60 seconds then repeat above exercises for 3 rounds.			
Dumbbell bi-cep curl and shoulder press	10	3	1 min
Push ups	12	3	1 min
Bent over dumbbell arm row	12	3	1 min
Rest 60 seconds then repeat above exercises for 3 rounds.			

Body weight and strength training

Week 6 Day 3

Exercise	Reps	Sets	Rest
T-Bend	10	3	1 min
Step ups with dumbbells	12 per side	3	1 min
Elbow or straight arm plank	75 seconds	3	1 min
Rest 60 seconds then repeat above exercises for 3 rounds.			
One arm dumbbell row	10 per side	3	1 min
Dumbbell bicep curl and shoulder press	10	3	1 min
Push ups	12	3	1 min
Rest 60 seconds then repeat above exercises for 3 rounds.			
Curtsy lunge (with dumbbells)	10 per side	3	1 min
Goblet squat with dumbbell	10	3	1 min
Mountain climbers	12 per side	3	1 min
Rest 60 seconds then repeat above exercises for 3 rounds.			

Body weight and strength training

Week 7 Day 1

Exercise	Reps	Sets	Rest
Push ups	12	3	1 min
Bulgarian split squat (use a bench or chair)	10	3	1 min
Mountain climbers	12 per side	3	1 min
Rest 60 seconds then repeat above exercises for 3 rounds.			
Dumbbell arm row and kickback	10	3	1 min
Goblet squat with dumbbell	10	3	1 min
One leg get ups (use a bench or chair)	10 per side	3	1 min
Rest 60 seconds then repeat above exercises for 3 rounds.			
Dumbbell bicep curl and shoulder press	10	3	1 min
T-Bend	10 per side	3	1 min
Russian Twist (with or without weight)	12 per side	3	1 min
Rest 60 seconds then repeat above exercises for 3 rounds.			

Body weight and strength training

Week 7 Day 2

Exercise	Reps	Sets	Rest
T-Bend	10	3	1 min
Dumbbell row and kickback	10	3	1 min
Bulgarian split squat (use a bench or chair)	10 per side	3	1 min
Rest 60 seconds then repeat above exercises for 3 rounds.			
Step ups and with dumbbells	10 per side	3	1 min
Tri-cep dips or overhead tri-cep extensions with dumbbells	12	3	1 min
Stiffleg deadlift (use a bench or chair)	10	3	1 min
Rest 60 seconds then repeat above exercises for 3 rounds.			
Mountain climbers	12 per side	3	1 min
Dumbbell hammer curl & bicep curl	10 each	3	1 min
Goblet squat with dumbbell	12	3	1 min
Rest 60 seconds then repeat above exercises for 3 rounds.			

Body weight and strength training

Week 7 Day 3

Exercise	Reps	Sets	Rest
Goblet squat with dumbbell	12	3	1 min
V-Ups	12	3	1 min
Tri-cep dips or overhead tri-cep extensions with dumbbells	12	3	1 min
Rest 60 seconds then repeat above exercises for 3 rounds.			
Stiff leg deadlifts (with barbell or dumbbells)	10	3	1 min
Elbow or straight arm plank	75 seconds	3	1 min
Dumbbell hammer curl & bicep curl	10 of each	3	1 min
Rest 60 seconds then repeat above exercises for 3 rounds.			
One arm dumbbell row	12 per side	3	1 min
One leg getups (use a bench or chair)	10 per side	3	1 min
T-Bend	10 per side	3	1 min
Rest 60 seconds then repeat above exercises for 3 rounds.			

Body weight and strength training

Week 8 Day 1

Exercise	Reps	Sets	Rest
Push ups	12	3	1 min
Curtsy lunge (with dumbbells)	12 per side	3	1 min
Step ups with dumbbells	12 per side	3	1 min
Bent over dumbbell row	12	3	1 min
V-Ups	12	3	1 min
Mountain climbers	12 per side	3	1 min
Dumbbell lateral arm raises	10	3	1 min
Goblet squat with dumbbell	12	3	1 min
Elbow or straight arm plank	80 seconds	3	1 min
Dumbbell Triple curl (hammer curl, bicep curl and reverse curl)	10 of each	3	1 min
Rest 60 seconds then repeat above exercises for 3 rounds.			

Body weight and strength training

Week 8 Day 2

Exercise	Reps	Sets	Rest
Curtsy lunge (with dumbbells)	12 per side	3	1 min
Lying cross over abdominal crunch	12 per side	3	1 min
Tri-cep dips or overhead tri-cep extensions with dumbbells	12	3	1 min
Walking lunges with dumbbells	12 per side	3	1 min
elbow or straight arm side planks	45 secs per side	3	1 min
Dumbbell Triple curl (hammer curl, bicep curl and reverse curl)	10 of each	3	1 min
Bent over dumbbell row with kickbacks	12	3	1 min
Goblet squat with dumbbell	12	3	1 min
One leg get ups (use a bench or chair)	12 per side	3	1 min
Lateral and front arm raises with dumbbells	12 per side	3	1 min
Rest 60 seconds then repeat above exercises for 3 rounds.			

Body weight and strength training

Week 8 Day 3

Exercise	Reps	Sets	Rest
Goblet squat	12	3	1 min
Tri-cep dips or overhead tri-cep extensions with dumbbells	12	3	1 min
Curtsy lunge (with dumbbells)	12 per side	3	1 min
Elbow or straight arm side plank	45 secs per side	3	1 min
Front and lateral arm raises with dumbbells	12 each	3	1 min
Bulgarian split squat (use a bench or chair)	12	3	1 min
V-ups	12	3	1 min
Alternating one arm dumbbell shoulder press	12 per side	3	1 min
Stiff leg deadlift wit a barbell or dumbbells	12	3	1 min
Rest 60 seconds then repeat above exercises for 3 rounds.			

Body weight and strength training

Week 9 Day 1

Exercise	Reps	Sets	Rest
Push ups	12	3	1 min
One leg get ups (use a bench or chair)	12 per side	3	1 min
Curtsy lunge (with dumbbells)	12 per side	3	1 min
Dumbbell shoulder press to French press	12	3	1 min
Goblet squat with dumbbell	12	3	1 min
Elbow or straight arm plank	80 seconds	3	1 min
One arm dumbbell row with kick back	12 per side	3	1 min
T-bend	12	3	1 min
Squat and lateral arm raise with dumbbells	12	3	1 min
Rest 60 seconds then repeat above exercises for 3 rounds.			

Body weight and strength training

Week 9 Day 2

Exercise	Reps	Sets	Rest
One leg get ups (use a bench or chair)	12 per side	3	1 min
Curtsy lunge with dumbbells	12 per side	3	1 min
Dumbbell bent over lateral arm raises	12	3	1 min
T-Bend	12	3	1 min
Lying crossover abdominal crunch	12 per side	3	1 min
One arm dumbbell row	12 per side	3	1 min
Dumbbell squat	12	3	1 min
Mountain climbers	15 per side	3	1 min
Dumbbell shoulder press and French press	12	3	1 min
Rest 60 seconds then repeat above exercises for 3 rounds.			

Body weight and strength training

Week 9 Day 3

Exercise	Reps	Sets	Rest
T-Bend	12 per side	3	1 min
Dumbbell shoulder press to French press	12	3	1 min
One leg get ups (use a bench or chair)	12 per side	3	1 min
Mountain climbers	15 per side	3	1 min
Push ups	12	3	1 min
Stiff leg deadlifts with a barbell or dumbbell	12	3	1 min
Russian twists with weights	15 per side	3	1 min
Bent over dumbbell row and kickback	12	3	1 min
Goblet squat with dumbbell	12	3	1 min
Rest 60 seconds then repeat above exercises for 3 rounds.			

Body weight and strength training

Week 10 Day 1

Exercise	Reps	Sets	Rest
Dumbbell front and lateral arm raises	12	3	1 min
Bent dumbbell row	12	3	1 min
Dumbbell shoulder press to French press	12	3	1 min
Rest 60 seconds then repeat above exercises for 3 rounds.			
Step ups with dumbbells	12 per side	3	1 min
Stiff leg deadlifts with a barbell or dumbbells	12	3	1 min
Goblet squats with dumbbell	12	3	1 min
Rest 60 seconds then repeat above exercises for 3 rounds.			
Ab wheel (roll forward, use the wall to stop, then roll back to starting position)	12	3	1 min
T-Bend	12	3	1 min
Mountain climbers	12 per side	3	1 min
Rest 60 seconds then repeat above exercises for 3 rounds.			

Body weight and strength training

Week 10 Day 2

Exercise	Reps	Sets	Rest
Dumbbell squat	12	3	1 min
Mountain climbers	12 per side	3	1 min
Stiff leg deadlifts with a barbell or dumbbell	12	3	1 min
Rest 60 seconds then repeat above exercises for 3 rounds.			
Step ups with dumbbells	12 per side	3	1 min
Ab wheel (roll forward,use the wall to stop, then roll back to starting position)	12	3	1 min
Elbow or straight arm plank	90 secs	3	1 min
Rest 60 seconds then repeat above exercises for 3 rounds.			
Dumbbell Triple curl (hammer curl, bicep curl and reverse curl)	12 each	3	1 min
Dumbbell shoulder press to tri-cep extension	12	3	1 min
Bent over arm row to kickbacks with dumbbells	12 per side	3	1 min
Rest 60 seconds then repeat above exercises for 3 rounds.			

Body weight and strength training

Week 10 Day 3

Exercise	Reps	Sets	Rest
Russian twists with weight	12 per side	3	1 min
Elbow or straight arm plank	90 seconds	3	1 min
Ab wheel (roll forward,use the wall to stop, then roll back to starting position)	12	3	1 min
Rest 60 seconds then repeat above exercises for 3 rounds.			
One arm dumbbell row	12 per side	3	1 min
Shoulder press with dumbbells	12	3	1 min
Dumbbell Triple curl (hammer curl, bicep curl and reverse curl)	12	3	1 min
Rest 60 seconds then repeat above exercises for 3 rounds.			
Stiff leg deadlift with a barbell or dumbbells	12	3	1 min
Dumbbell squat	12	3	1 min
One leg get ups (use a bench or chair)	12 per side	3	1 min
Rest 60 seconds then repeat above exercises for 3 rounds.			

Body weight and strength training

Week 11 Day 1

Exercise	Reps	Sets	Rest
Dumbbell shoulder press to French press	12	3	1 min
Curtsy lunges with dumbbells	12 per side	3	1 min
Bulgarian split squat with dumbbells	12 per side	3	1 min
Rest 60 seconds then repeat above exercises for 3 rounds.			
Bent over dumbbell arm rows to kickback	12	3	1 min
V-ups	15	3	1 min
Elbow or straight arm plank	90 seconds	3	1 min
Rest 60 seconds then repeat above exercises for 3 rounds.			
Pullover to tricep extension with one dumbbell	12	3	1 min
T-Bend	12	3	1 min
Ab wheel (roll forward,use the wall to stop, then roll back to starting position)	15	3	1 min
Rest 60 seconds then repeat above exercises for 3 rounds.			

Body weight and strength training

Week 11 Day 2

Exercise	Reps	Sets	Rest
T-bend	12 per side	3	1 min
Bent over dumbbell arm row to kickback	12	3	1 min
V-ups	15	3	1 min
Rest 60 seconds then repeat above exercises for 3 rounds.			
Elbow or straight arm plank	90 seconds	3	1 min
Dumbbell Triple curl (hammer curl, bicep curl and reverse curl)	10 of each	3	1 min
Stiff leg deadlifts with a barbell or dumbbells	12	3	1 min
Rest 60 seconds then repeat above exercises for 3 rounds.			
Bulgarian split squat with dumbbells	12 per side	3	1 min
Pullover to tri-cep extension with one dumbbell	12	3	1 min
Walking lunge with dumbbells	12 per side	3	1 min
Rest 60 seconds then repeat above exercises for 3 rounds.			

Body weight and strength training

Week 11 Day 3

Exercise	Reps	Sets	Rest
One leg get ups (use a bench or chair)	12 per side	3	1 min
Curtsy lunge with dumbbells	12 per side	3	1 min
Tri-cep dips or overhead tri-cep extensions with dumbbells	15	3	1 min
Rest 60 seconds then repeat above exercises for 3 rounds.			
Stiff leg deadlifts with barbell or dumbbells	12	3	1 min
Elbow or straight arm plank	90 seconds	3	1 min
Dumbbell Triple curl (hammer curl, bicep curl and reverse curl)	10 of each	3	1 min
Rest 60 seconds then repeat above exercises for 3 rounds.			
Mountain climbers	15 per side	3	1 min
T-Bend	12 per side	3	1 min
One arm dumbbell shoulder press	12 per side	3	1 min
Rest 60 seconds then repeat above exercises for 3 rounds.			

Body weight and strength training

Week 12 Day 1

Exercise	Reps	Sets	Rest
One arm dumbbell row	12 per side	3	1 min
Stiff leg deadlift (with barbell or dumbbells)	12	3	1 min
Bulgarian split squat with dumbbells	12 per side	3	1 min
Shoulder press and French press with barbell or dumbbells	12	3	1 min
One leg get ups (use a bench or chair)	12 per side	3	1 min
Dumbbell Triple curl (hammer curl, bicep curl and reverse curl)	10 of each	3	1 min
Alternate dumbbell shoulder press	12 per side	3	1 min
Step ups with dumbbells	12	3	1 min
Elbow or straight arm plank	90 seconds	3	1 min
Rest 60 seconds then repeat above exercises for 3 rounds.			

Body weight and strength training

Week 12 Day 2

Exercise	Reps	Sets	Rest
Stiff leg deadlift (with barbell or dumbbells)	12	3	1 min
Dumbbell squat and lateral arm raise	12	3	1 min
Dumbbell straight arm pullover to tri-cep extension	12	3	1 min
Step ups with dumbbells	12	3	1 min
Ab wheel (roll forward,use the wall to stop, then roll back to starting position)	15	3	1 min
Dumbbell shoulder press and French press	12	3	1 min
V-ups	12	3	1 min
Bulgarian split squat with dumbbells	12 per side	3	1 min
Dumbbell Triple curl (hammer curl, bicep curl and reverse curl)	10 of each	3	1 min
Rest 60 seconds then repeat above exercises for 3 rounds.			

Body weight and strength training

Week 12 Day 3

Exercise	Reps	Sets	Rest
Curtsy lunge with dumbbells	15 per side	3	1 min
Straight arm Pullover to tri-cep extension	12	3	1 min
Stiff leg deadlift (use a bench or chair)	12	3	1 min
Ab wheel (roll forward,use the wall to stop, then roll back to starting position)	15	3	1 min
Alternate dumbbell press	15 per side	3	1 min
Walking lunges with dumbbells	12 per side	3	1 min
Dumbbell squat and lateral raise	12	3	1 min
Dumbbell shoulder press to tri-cep extension	12	3	1 min
T-Bend	12 per side	3	1 min
Rest 60 seconds then repeat above exercises for 3 rounds.			

Well done! You have completed the whole 12 weeks.

How do you feel? Stronger, more confident, sexier?

Can you see any changes in your body composition? As I said earlier in the program…don't worry about what the scale says, muscle weighs more than fat, so while you have lost body fat you have built lean muscle. Your clothes might fit better, feel looser yet the scale says you weigh more or it has stayed the same. This is quite normal. Throw the scale away and go by what your measurements say instead.

Are you ready to start over? If you do start over, start with the amount of reps you finished off with or increase your sets to 4 and start with the same amount of reps given in the program. Alternatively, start with the same reps and sets in the program but increase your weights.

Please do contact me if you have any questions that I can help you with. I would love to hear about your progress, the obstacles you encounter and anything you would like to share with me regarding your fitness journey. I have not started a group or blog yet as this is a very new creation of mine but I will be sure to you let you know once I have a big enough fan base.

My e-mail is ellieg.workouts.sa@gmail.com

I hope you have had a great time doing this program. I had a great time creating it. There are more programs to come in the future. Keep your eyes on Amazon.com

May your days be full of health, wealth and happiness!

Until next time.

EllieG ☺

www.ingramcontent.com/pod-product-compliance
Lightning Source LLC
Chambersburg PA
CBHW040050240726
48664CB00004B/1136